RESPIRATORY SYNCYTIAL VIRUS IN ADULTS

REMEDY GUIDE FOR RESPIRATORY SYNCYTIAL VIRUS IN ADULTS

DR. J. WALLER

Contents

INTRODUCTION 3

CHAPTER ONE 6

Risk and Transmission Factors 6

Adult Symptoms and Signs...10

Diagnosis and Assessment 13

Adult Prevention Techniques...17

CHAPTER TWO 22

Adult Treatment Strategies...22

High-Risk Adult Demographics...26

Adult Complications and Long-Term Impacts 29

CHAPTER THREE 32

Enhanced Vulnerability to Additional Infections....................32

Emotional Health and Coping Mechanisms 34

Get rest and give self-care priority: 35

CONCLUSION...38

THE END 42

INTRODUCTION

Although it is frequently linked to illnesses in newborns and early children, adults can also contract Respiratory Syncytial Virus (RSV). An overview of RSV in adults is provided here:

A common respiratory virus that can infect the lungs and respiratory tract is called the Respiratory Syncytial Virus (RSV). RSV infections can happen to people of any age, including adults, despite being the most common cause of respiratory disorders in children. Even though RSV infections in adults are often less severe than in babies, they can nevertheless cause serious respiratory problems.

Severe RSV infections may be more common in adults, particularly in the elderly, those with compromised immune systems, and people with underlying medical disorders. Adults with common symptoms include sore throats, sneezing, coughing, and nasal congestion. RSV can cause pneumonia or bronchitis in more severe cases.

When an infected individual coughs or sneezes, respiratory droplets are the main way that the virus is disseminated. Additionally, it can be acquired by touching the face after coming into contact with an infected surface or object.

Adult RSV transmission can be decreased by taking preventive steps such frequent hand washing, avoiding direct contact with sick people, and adopting respiratory etiquette. Supportive care and symptom control are crucial in assisting people in recovering from RSV infection, even though there isn't a specific antiviral medication for the illness.

Adults should be aware of RSV symptoms, seek medical assistance when necessary, and take precautions to stop the virus from spreading, especially if they belong to high-risk groups.

CHAPTER ONE

Risk and Transmission Factors

Adults who cough or sneeze with an infected individual can spread the respiratory syncytial virus (RSV) by respiratory droplets. The following are some important details about adult RSV transmission and risk factors:

Breathing Droplets:

RSV is a highly infectious virus that is mostly transmitted by respiratory droplets that are released into the atmosphere when an infected person sneezes, coughs, or talks. People in close proximity may inhale these droplets and become infected.

Direct Communication:

Direct contact with an infected individual or surfaces contaminated with the virus can also result in the transmission of RSV. Transmission can occur when the virus comes into contact with a surface or object and then comes into contact with the face, particularly the mouth, nose, or eyes.

Communal Environments:

Adults who live in crowded environments, like homes, long-term care institutions, and healthcare facilities, are more likely to contract RSV. In these settings, the virus is more likely to spread through close contact.

Reduced Immune Responses:

Adults who take immunosuppressive medicines, are elderly, have underlying medical disorders, or otherwise have compromised immune systems are more vulnerable to severe RSV infections.

Long-Term Medical Conditions:

Severe RSV infections may be more common in those with long-term medical illnesses such as diabetes, heart disease, chronic obstructive pulmonary disease (COPD), or other respiratory disorders.

Age:

Although severe RSV infections are more common in newborns, aging-related immune system alterations also put older adults at risk for problems.

Exposure at Work:

Workers in some professions that have frequent interaction with the public, including healthcare professionals, may be more susceptible to RSV exposure.

Adults can prevent infections by washing their hands frequently, avoiding direct contact with sick people, and keeping their surroundings clean. RSV vaccines are presently being developed, but as of my most recent knowledge update in January 2022, adult access to them might be restricted.

Reducing the spread and effects of RSV in adults requires adherence to preventive measures, early symptom recognition, and awareness of risk factors.

Adult Symptoms and Signs

Adults infected with the respiratory syncytial virus (RSV) may present with a variety of symptoms, varying in intensity. The following are some typical indications and symptoms of adult RSV:

Symptoms of Upper Respiratory:

Similar to symptoms of a normal cold, nasal congestion and runny nose are common early symptoms of RSV in adults.

Cough

One of the main signs of RSV is persistent coughing. The cough may begin lightly and progressively worsen.

Throat Pain:

Throat irritation or pain is another typical symptom.

Temperature spike:

Fever is possible in adults with RSV infections, though it might vary in intensity.

Breathiness Shortness:

Breathing difficulties or shortness of breath may occur in certain people, particularly in more severe situations.

Sighing:

Certain individuals infected with RSV may exhibit wheezing, a high-pitched whistling sound made during breathing.

Weary:

Fatigue and generalized weakness are prevalent symptoms that lower general energy levels.

Physical Pains:

There could be soreness and muscle aches all over the body.

Headache:

One symptom that some individuals with RSV may have is headaches.

It's vital to remember that adult RSV symptoms might overlap with those of other respiratory illnesses, making a diagnosis based only on symptoms difficult. Adult RSV infections can occasionally be less severe than those in newborns and early children.

While the majority of adults who contract RSV do so without any problems, those who already have underlying medical disorders or compromised immune systems may be more susceptible to a serious infection. It is best to seek medical assistance for appropriate examination and management if you suspect an RSV infection or if your symptoms are severe.

Diagnosis and Assessment

Adult instances of Respiratory Syncytial Virus (RSV) diagnosis are made using a combination of laboratory tests and clinical examination. The following is how medical practitioners might handle the diagnosis and assessment of RSV in adults:

Clinical Assessment:

Medical History: The physician will ask about the patient's symptoms, including when the respiratory symptoms started and how they progressed, as well as any possible contacts with sick people.

Physical Examination: To evaluate respiratory symptoms such coughing, wheezing, and shortness of breath, a comprehensive physical examination may be carried out.

Laboratory Examinations:

Throat or Nasal Swab: A sample of the nose or throat may be taken with a swab for laboratory analysis. To find out if RSV genetic material is present, the most popular techniques are polymerase chain reaction (PCR) assays or fast antigen tests.

Blood Examinations:

A blood sample may be drawn in some circumstances to screen for the presence of RSV antibodies, while swab tests are more frequently utilized in blood tests.

Chest X-ray:

To evaluate lung involvement and rule out illnesses like pneumonia, a chest X-ray may be used if the respiratory symptoms are severe or if consequences are predicted.

Tests for Pulmonary Function:

To evaluate lung function in people exhibiting severe respiratory distress, pulmonary function tests could be carried out.

It's crucial to remember that, particularly in mild cases, laboratory testing may not necessarily be required for the diagnosis of RSV in adults. When diagnosing a patient, clinical symptoms and medical history are frequently important factors to consider.

It is imperative to get medical assistance as soon as possible if symptoms seem severe or if you suspect an RSV infection. Appropriate management, such as supportive care, symptom alleviation, and monitoring for consequences, is made possible by an early diagnosis.

Adult Prevention Techniques

Adults can prevent Respiratory Syncytial Virus (RSV) by implementing a number of preventative measures that lower the likelihood of exposure and transmission. The following are some adult preventive techniques:

Hand Sanitization:

Hands should be periodically washed for at least 20 seconds with soap and water, especially after interacting with ill people, touching surfaces, or being in public.

When soap and water are not easily accessible, use hand sanitizers with alcohol basis.

Steer clear of close contact:

Reduce your close contact with sick people, especially if they have respiratory problems.

Keep a safe distance from people who appear ill and practice social distancing in busy areas.

Pneumonia Etiquette:

When you sneeze or cough, cover your mouth and nose with your elbow or a tissue.

Once tissues have been properly disposed of, wash your hands right away.

Empty and Rinse:

Make sure to routinely clean and sanitize frequently touched areas in your home and place of business, like light switches, doorknobs, and electronics.

Remain Up to Date:

Remain aware of regional outbreaks and use caution, particularly during the height of the RSV season.

Immunization (if accessible):

Although there isn't yet a widely accessible adult RSV vaccination, keep up with developments about RSV vaccine development and talk through your alternatives with your healthcare physician.

Boost Your Immune System:

Eating a balanced diet, exercising frequently, getting enough sleep, and managing stress are all important components of a healthy lifestyle. Having a robust immune system can aid in avoiding illnesses.

Don't Touch Your Face:

Refrain from touching your face, particularly your lips, nose, or eyes, since this can facilitate the transmission of respiratory viruses.

If You're Sick, Stay at Home:

To stop the sickness from spreading to others, stay home from work or social events if you have respiratory symptoms or are feeling under the weather.

Precautionary Steps at Work:

Whenever feasible, try to work from home while the activity of respiratory viruses is high.

Companies might put in place rules to encourage workers who are ill to stay at home and to foster a tidy workplace.

The risk of RSV and other respiratory infections in adults can be significantly decreased by using these preventative measures. Proactively maintaining proper hygiene and implementing preventative measures contributes to community and individual protection.

CHAPTER TWO

Adult Treatment Strategies

Adults with Respiratory Syncytial Virus (RSV) infections are treated mostly with supportive care because no particular antiviral drug is approved for RSV infections in this age range. The following are some typical methods for treating RSV in adults:

Symptomatic Management:

Fever, congestion in the nose, coughing, and other symptoms can be treated with over-the-counter drugs. It is crucial, therefore, that these drugs be taken under a doctor's supervision.

Control of Pain and Fever:

To manage pain and lower temperature, acetaminophen or nonsteroidal anti-inflammatory medications (NSAIDs) may be prescribed.

Fluid Consumption:

It's important to make sure you're getting enough fluids to avoid dehydration, even if you're not feeling very hungry.

Relax:

Resting well enables the body to concentrate its efforts on combating the infection.

Air that has been humidified:

Breathing can be made easier and nasal congestion can be reduced by using a humidifier.

bronchodilators:

Bronchodilators may be administered to treat wheezing or bronchospasm in order to enhance airflow.

Treatment using Oxygen:

Supplementary oxygen therapy could be required in extreme situations if there is a great deal of respiratory distress.

Inpatient care (if necessary):

Serious instances of RSV in adults may necessitate hospitalization for close observation and supportive care, especially in those with weakened immune systems or underlying medical disorders.

It's crucial to remember that viruses like RSV cannot be treated with drugs. The goals of treatment are supportive care and symptom management.

To lower the risk of RSV transmission in adults, preventive steps are crucial. These include maintaining a clean environment, avoiding direct contact with sick people, and practicing good hand hygiene.

Getting medical help is advised if a person thinks they may have RSV or if their symptoms are severe. Medical experts can offer pertinent advice and decide on the best course of action based on the patient's general health and the severity of their symptoms.

Some adult groups are thought to be more vulnerable to serious consequences resulting from infections with the respiratory syncytial virus (RSV). Among these at-risk demographics are:

Senior Citizens:

Due to immune system alterations brought on by aging, adults 65 years of age and older have a higher chance of developing severe RSV infections.

Those with Coexisting Medical Conditions:

Severe RSV infections are more common in adults with long-term medical disorders like asthma, diabetes, cardiovascular disease, chronic obstructive pulmonary disease (COPD), or weakened immune systems.

Those with impaired immune systems:

Severe RSV infections are more common in people with compromised immune systems, whether as a result of illnesses like HIV/AIDS or immunosuppressive drugs like post-transplant.

People residing in extended-care facilities:

Due to shared facilities and close quarters, residents of nursing homes and long-term care facilities may be more vulnerable.

Healthcare Professionals:

Healthcare workers are more likely to be exposed to RSV than other workers, particularly those who operate in environments where they can come into touch with respiratory diseases.

Smokers:

Smokers may have weakened respiratory systems, which increases their vulnerability to respiratory diseases like RSV.

People Affected by Neuromuscular Disorders:

Respiratory muscle weakness may put those with neuromuscular illnesses, such muscular dystrophy, at higher risk of consequences.

Expectant Mothers:

The immune system changes during pregnancy, which may affect how the body reacts to infections, even though pregnant people are not always more likely to have severe RSV infections.

For those in these high-risk groups, preventive steps are essential. These include vaccinations when available, practicing excellent hand hygiene, and avoiding close contact with sick people. Additionally, if respiratory sickness symptoms, particularly severe symptoms, appear in these people, immediate medical assistance is recommended.

Adult Complications and Long-Term Impacts

Although the majority of adult instances of Respiratory Syncytial Virus (RSV) are moderate and self-limiting, serious infections can result in complications and cause long-lasting damage in certain people. The following are possible long-term consequences and difficulties linked to RSV in adults:

bronchitis:

A bronchial tube inflammation known as bronchitis can result from severe RSV infections. Breathing difficulties, mucous production, and a chronic cough are possible outcomes of this.

Pneumonia:

RSV infections can occasionally lead to lung infections called pneumonia. Chest pain, a strong cough, and a high temperature are all possible signs of pneumonia.

Intensive Phase of Chronic Illnesses:

Adults who already have respiratory disorders, such as asthma or chronic obstructive pulmonary disease (COPD), may find that their symptoms worsen both during and after an RSV infection.

Breathing Problems:

Severe RSV infections can result in low oxygen levels, fast breathing, and dyspnea due to respiratory distress.

CHAPTER THREE

Bedding in:

A hospital stay may be necessary for some individuals with RSV, particularly those in high-risk categories, in order to get intensive monitoring and supportive care.

Enhanced Vulnerability to Additional Infections

RSV infections have the potential to impair immunity, increasing a person's susceptibility to further respiratory infections.

Symptoms of persistent respiratory failure:

While the majority of adults recover completely from RSV, some people may endure long-lasting respiratory symptoms such coughing and dyspnea.

It's crucial to remember that older folks, those with underlying medical issues, and those with compromised immune systems are more likely to experience serious consequences and long-term impacts. The majority of healthy adults recover from RSV without any lasting effects.

Reducing the risk of problems related to RSV requires early symptom assessment, preventive interventions, and rapid medical attention. People who have severe respiratory symptoms should consult a doctor so they can be properly evaluated and treated.

Emotional Health and Coping Mechanisms

It can be difficult to manage a respiratory disease like Respiratory Syncytial Virus (RSV) on both a physical and emotional level. The following coping mechanisms and advice can help adults with RSV maintain their emotional health:

Acknowledge Your Emotions:

Feeling a range of emotions, such as concern, anxiety, or annoyance, is normal. Accept and acknowledge these emotions without passing judgment.

Remain Up to Date:

Learn about RSV, its symptoms, and how the illness progresses. Being aware of what to anticipate might reduce anxiety.

Interact with Medical Professionals:

Keep lines of communication open and honest with your medical professional. Talk about your symptoms, available treatments, and any worries you may have.

Get rest and give self-care priority:

Give yourself enough time to relax and heal. Make self-care activities that improve your emotional and physical health a priority.

Seek Assistance:

Talk to loved ones, a support group, or friends about your feelings and worries. Expressing your feelings can be incredibly relieving at times.

Maintain Contact:

Maintain your relationships with your loved ones, even if they are virtual. A vital component of emotional health is social support.

Keep a Schedule:

Even if you're ill, create a daily schedule to give yourself structure and a sense of normalcy. Achievable yet modest aims might bring happiness.

Reduce the Overload of Information:

While it's important to keep informed, try to avoid spending too much time with news or health information that could make you anxious.

Use relaxation and mindfulness techniques:

To reduce tension and encourage relaxation, try mindfulness exercises, deep breathing techniques, or meditation.

Emphasize the Positive:

Focus on the good things in your life and the achievements you've made toward healing. Honor modest accomplishments.

Request Assistance:

Never be afraid to seek friends, family, or medical experts for assistance if you need it. There are several ways to get support.

Keep in mind that coping mechanisms might differ from person to person, so it's critical to determine which ones are most effective for you. Consider getting help from a mental health professional if you continue to experience anxiety or distress. They may offer you coping mechanisms and assistance that are specific to your needs.

CONCLUSION

In conclusion, adults may contract respiratory infections caused by the Respiratory Syncytial Virus (RSV), which can cause mild to severe symptoms. RSV can be dangerous for some adult populations, especially those with compromised immune systems, underlying medical disorders, or senior age, even though it is frequently linked to infections in newborns.

A clean environment, avoiding direct contact with sick people, and practicing good hand hygiene are all important preventive strategies that can lower the risk of RSV transmission in adults. Although there isn't a specific antiviral treatment for RSV in adults, managing symptoms and providing supportive care are crucial parts of the overall recovery strategy.

RSV infections can cause more serious side effects in high-risk groups, such as the elderly and people with long-term medical issues. Thus, early intervention depends on receiving medical attention as soon as possible and being vigilant about identifying signs.

In order to effectively manage RSV emotionally, one must recognize and deal with any sentiments of worry or annoyance as well as enlist the help of friends, family, and medical professionals. Throughout the healing process, keeping a healthy lifestyle, giving self-care first priority, and remaining educated about the illness all contribute to overall well-being.

Ongoing attempts to comprehend RSV in adults, create prevention measures, and investigate prospective treatments will help to more effectively manage this respiratory virus in the adult population as long as research and medical developments continue.

THE END